GOING VEGAN

The Ideal Cookbook of Tasty Meals to Prepare for Vegan Foodies

The Health Buff

Table Of Contents

The Vegan Diet

The Vegan Diet has indeed become more popular nowadays. A great number of people has dared to try and loved it. In fact, there are also some who has become advocates of this diet. There are reasons why people seem to love consuming food the vegan way, some of which are: health, ethical, or environmental reasons. But what is really a Vegan Diet?

Basically, the vegan diet is a diet which does not involve the consumption of any animal products, and yes, we're talking about meat, eggs, and dairy too. Going for the vegan diet means you can only consume plants – such as green leafy vegetables, fruits, nuts, and grains.

People go for this diet as this is known to help one lose weight and achieve a lower body mass index – that is, if you're doing it right. Not only does it help in achieving the close-to-perfect bod, it also makes one become healthier if the diet is planned accordingly.

The Vegan Variety

Being a vegan does not only mean getting rid of products made from animals, in fact, as the vegan diet becomes a trend, it was broken down in different categories. Here are some of the common types of the vegan diet:

80/10/10

This vegan diet gets its name from the goal of getting 80% of calories from carbohydrates like raw fruits, 10% from raw, plant-based protein, and 10% fat raw food. It is also known to be the 811rv or LFRV which stands for Low-Fat, Raw-Food. The 80/10/10 vegan diet is said to be a long-term resolution to intensify longevity and lessen disease and obesity.

Junk-Food Vegan Diet

Nope, it's not that junk food that you would probably binge on while watching a movie – chips, pizza, popcorns, the list goes on. Instead, this vegan diet is known to be such because there are vegans who choose to chow down highly-processed foods which are oftentimes found on groceries and convenience stores. This not-so-advisable vegan diet lacks in whole plant foods and relies too much on mock meats, variety of cheese, fries, vegan desserts, and the like.

Raw-Food Vegan Diet

This category of the vegan diet is also known as raw foodism or raw veganism. It basically allows people who practice it to only munch on completely raw and unprocessed foods. The basis of the rawness of the food for this diet is, the food should have never been heat for more than 104-118 F or 40-48C. More so, the food should also not be refined, treated with pesticides, pasteurized, or processed in any way. Nevertheless, you can prepare food by blending, dehydrating, juicing, soaking, and sprouting.

Raw 'til 4

This vegan diet is more known to be a lifestyle rather than a diet since it also requires high-energy exercise. The focus of this diet is to brush aside calorie restriction and welcome the act of eating and living plentifully. That 4 in its name is not there for nothing. Four means you can only eat raw fruits and greens until 4PM while having the option of a cooked plant-based meal for dinner.

The Starch

Solution. This diet is made famous by Dr. John McDougall who believes that there is a specific diet to support the health of every animal at its best. For humans, that would be based on starches. Hence, the solution... or the diet. This low-fat, high-carb vegan diet is likely similar with the 80/10/10 diet but the difference is this diet mainly focuses on cooked starches such as rice, corn, potatoes, and beans instead of fruits.

Whole-food Vegan Diet

This vegan diet pretty much allows a vegan practice following a whole food diet that is based on a great variety of whole plant foods like vegetables, fruits, nuts, seeds, legumes, and whole grains.

Why Go Vegan?

There is no doubt why the number of people who go for the vegan diet continually increase. There are a number of reasons why it's beneficial to go vegan. Let's get this list started, shall we?

Because we love mother Earth

So basically, recycling is one of the mainstream ways to save the Earth. But how is being vegan connected to recycling? Producing meat and other animal products creates a freight on the environment. Here's how: we use crops, water, and other means to transport to produce such products. These materials used for these allows people to deforest, use more fuel, air-polluting factories in some cases to produce feeds for animals. More so, did you know that raising animals to be only devoured in the end actually produces more greenhouse gas emissions compared to cars, planes, and other forms of transportation? We are all aware how much greenhouse affects the earth. Bottomline: Going vegan allows the decrease of deforestation, pollution, and greenhouse gas emission, and it increases the chances of saving water and other earthly resources.

Because we sympathize with animals

Don't you just feel bad for the cows and pigs that are killed just for us to have something to guzzle? Animals too are living beings that have the right to live and be free just like humans. Protecting and respecting the lives of animals are just some of the reasons why people opt to go vegan instead. More so, this could also mean, them, supporting animal rights.

Because we care for the people

Going for a plant-based style of living is a more sustainable way of feeding a human family. It only requires one third of the land needed to support meat and dairy diet. Given the global issues on unstable supply of food and water that continually hit other countries, this is the best time to start the vegan way of living.

Because our health is important

This is most probably the major reason why people are in dire to fully practice being a vegan – for its health benefits. Increased energy, younger looking skin, everlasting youth – these are just some of the claims of the people who practice veganism. Who would not want that anyway? Other that the physical contributions the vegan diet can bring humans, this diet also contributes to our well-being in general. A well-planned vegan diet gives us protein, iron, calcium, and pretty much other important vitamins and minerals our body needs. It decreases the chances of us having obesity, heart disease, cancer, and diabetes.

Sure, there are other reasons to go be the best vegan out there! But pretty much sure you're now excited to try out some mouth-watering recipes to start your journey to the vegan diet. So here are some recipes for you to enjoy and continue practicing the art of veganism.

Mouthwatering Vegan Recipes

Bean and Rice Soup

What you need:
- 1 small green bell pepper
- 1 small red bell pepper
- 1 tbsp sunflower oil
- 1 medium onion
- 1 tbsp tomato puree
- 1 (15-oz) can coconut milk
- ½ cup long-grain rice
- 1 (15-oz) can red kidney beans
- 2 garlic cloves
- 2 stalks celery
- 2 carrots
- 2 bay leaves
- 2 - 2 1/2 tsp dried thyme
- 2 tbsp olive oil
- 3 cups tomato juice
- 3 cups vegetable bouillon
- 3 cups day-old bread cubes
- 4 tsp paprika
- sea salt and black pepper for the croutons

What to do first:
- Seed and chop the green and the red bell peppers
- Chop the onion, celery stalks, and carrots
- Mince the garlic cloves

Now for the main dish:
- Heat the oil in a large saucepan and add the onion and cook over medium-high heat for 5–7 minutes until the onion is soft
- Add the garlic, celery, carrots, peppers, bay leaves, and 2 teaspoons of paprika, and cook for another 5 minutes
- Combine in the tomato juice, tomato paste and thyme leaves, then cook for 5 minutes
- Add the bouillon, coconut milk, and rice
- Bring to a boil, reduce the heat, cover, and simmer for 30 minutes
- Add the kidney beans and cook for another 15 minutes
- Remove the bay leaves and season to taste with salt and pepper before serving garnished with croutons.

For the croutons:
- Toss the cubes of stale bread with the following:
- olive oil
- 2 teaspoons of paprika
- thyme
- Next, spread in a single layer on a baking sheet
- Bake at 375°F for 4–5 minutes until golden brown

Sweet Potato Soup

What you need:
- 1 onion
- 1 tbsp fresh ginger
- 1 tbsp vegan Thai red curry paste
- 1 tsp salt
- 1 litre / 1¾ pints vegan stock
- 1 lime
- 2 tsp vegetable oil
- 660g /1 lb 7 oz sweet potatoes
- 400ml / 14 fl oz canned reduced-fat coconut milk
- 30g / 1 oz finely chopped fresh coriander, to garnish

What to do first:
- Dice the onion and sweet potatoes
- Chop the ginger finely
- Juice the lime

Now for the main dish:
- Heat the oil over a medium–high heat in a large, heavy-based saucepan
- Add the onion and ginger and cook and stir for about 5 minutes or until soft
- Add the curry paste and salt and cook, stir for a further minute or so
- Add the sweet potatoes, coconut milk and stock and bring to the boil
- Reduce the heat to medium and simmer, uncovered, for about 20 minutes or until the sweet potatoes are soft
- Purée the soup, either in batches in a blender or food processor or using a hand-held blender
- Return the soup to the heat and bring back up to a simmer

- Stir in the lime juice just before serving
- Serve hot and garnished with coriander

Turmeric Tomato Soup

What you need:
*   1/2 teaspoon of turmeric
*   1 can of coconut milk
*   2 cloves garlic
*   3 large peeled tomatoes
*   Sea salt and black pepper to taste

What to do first:
*   Mince garlic cloves
*   Peel tomatoes

Here's what to do:
*   Blend. Heat. Serve!

Crunchy Tofu Bowl

What you need:
*   1/4 c. red wine vinegar
*   1/4 c. Thai sweet chili sauce
*   1/2 small red onion
*   1 tbsp. olive oil
*   1 seedless cucumber
*   1 c. cooked quinoa
*   2 tbsp. vegetable oil
*   2 tbsp. roasted cashew halves
*   3 tbsp. cornstarch
*   14 oz. extra-firm tofu
*   Parsley leaves for garnish

What to do first:
*   Slice the tofu 1/4 inch thick
*   Slice the red onion thinly

- Chop the cucumber

Now for the main dish:
- Place on cutting board between paper towels; top it off with a baking sheet and again, top it off with large cans or other weight
- Let it stand for around 10 minutes
- Soak red onion in cold water
- Combine red wine vinegar and Thai sweet chili sauce, olive oil and 1/4 teaspoon salt
- Pat the onion to dry; toss with half of vinaigrette and cucumber
- Sprinkle tofu on both sides with cornstarch
- In a 12-inch skillet, heat vegetable oil on medium-high until hot
- Carefully add the tofu
- Cook until deep golden brown, 2 to 3 minutes per side
- Drain on paper towels.
- Divide quinoa among 4 bowls
- Finally, top each with salad, roasted cashew halves, parsley leaves and tofu

Vegan Pesto Pasta

What you need:
* 1/4 c. packed fresh parsley
* 1/2 c. store-bought refrigerated pesto
* 1 lb. spaghetti
* 1 medium yellow squash
* 1 medium zucchini
* 1 small bell pepper
* 1 lemon
* 1 pt. grape tomatoes
* 2 ears of shucked corn
* 2 tbsp. olive oil
* 4 green onions

What to do first:
* Chop the fresh parsley
* Cut the squash and zucchini into ½" thick slices
* Seed the small bell pepper and cut into sixths
* Slice the grape tomatoes in half
* Shuck two ears of corn
* Trim the onions

Now for the main dish:
* Heat grill on medium-high. Cook spaghetti as label directs
* Rinse, drain well, and let cool completely the cooked spaghetti
* Toss corn, squash, zucchini, bell pepper and onions with oil and 1/2 teaspoon each salt and black pepper until well coated in large bowl
* Grill the corn, turning them every 10 minutes or until charred in spots

- Grill the squash, zucchini, and bell pepper for around 4 to 6 minutes or until tender and grill marks appear, turning once
- Grill the onions for 2 minutes or until tender and slightly charred, turning occasionally
- Grate 1/2 teaspoon zest and squeeze 2 tablespoons juice from the lemon
- Blend in the pesto and 1/2 teaspoon each salt and pepper – all in a large bowl
- Chop the squash, zucchini, pepper and onions then add to bowl with pesto
- Cut the kernels from cobs and add to bowl along with tomatoes, parsley and cooked pasta
- Toss to combine and serve at room temperature

Avocado, Beet, and Mushroom Salad

What you need:
- 1/4 c. lemon juice
- 1 small shallot
- 2 ripe avocados
- 2 sheets matzo
- 3 tbsp. olive oil
- 4 medium portobello mushroom caps
- 5 oz. baby kale
- 8 oz. precooked beets

What to do first:
- Chop the precooked beets and the small shallots finely
- Slice ripe avocados thinly
- Crush matzo into bite-size pieces

Now for the main dish:
- Spray portobello mushroom caps with nonstick cooking spray and sprinkle with 1/2 teaspoon salt on a large rimmed baking sheet
- Roast at 450°F 20 minutes or until tender
- Whisk the lemon juice, olive oil, shallot and 1/4 teaspoon each salt and pepper
- Toss half with baby kale and beets
- Divide among serving plates
- Top with avocados, matzo, and portobellos, all thinly sliced
- Serve with remaining dressing on the side

Spring Minestrone

What you need:
- 1 bunch asparagus
- 1 can (15 oz.) navy beans
- 1 medium leek
- 2 tbsp. olive oil
- 2 medium carrots
- 2 qt. lower-sodium vegetable or chicken broth
- 2 tbsp. fresh dill
- 3 large red potatoes
- 8 sprigs fresh thyme

What to do first:
- Slice the asparagus
- Rinse and drain (optional) the navy beans
- Slice the leek thinly
- Chop the fresh dill, red potatoes
- Tie together fresh thyme

Now for the main dish:
- Heat 2 tablespoons olive oil on medium in an 8-quart saucepot
- Add the carrots, leek, fresh thyme, and 1/4 teaspoon salt
- Cook for 8 minutes stir continuously
- Add the red potatoes, chopped, and lower-sodium vegetable or chicken broth. Partially cover and heat to boiling on high and reduce heat to simmer
- Cook 25 minutes or until potatoes are tender
- Add asparagus and simmer for 3 minutes or until it is tender. Discard thyme
- Add in the fresh dill, navy beans (optional), 1/2 teaspoon pepper, and 1/4 teaspoon salt

No Bake Choco-Cherry Supercarb Bars

What you need:
- 1/3 c. honey
- 1/2 c. quinoa
- 1/2 c. chia seeds
- 1/2 c. sliced almonds
- 1/2 c. dried cherries
- 1/2 c. chopped dark chocolate
- 1/2 c. pureed prunes (from about 1 c. prunes)
- 3/4 c. creamy almond butter
- 2 tbsp. coconut oil
- 2 c. old-fashioned oats

Here's what to do:
- Line a large baking sheet with parchment paper
- Combine the following in a large bowl: almonds, cherries, chia seeds, chocolate, oats, and quinoa
- Heat the almond butter, honey, coconut oil, and add 1/2 teaspoon salt until melted and smooth. Stir it occasionally in a small saucepan on low heat. Add in prune puree.
- Surge the almond butter mixture over the oat mixture and combine by stir
- Form into bars using about 1/3 cup mixture for each using hands
- Place on prepared sheet and refrigerate until set, about 1 hour
- Store in refrigerator in an airtight container

Mushroom-Quinoa Burger

What you need:
- For Burgers
- 1/4 c. red onion
- 1/2 c. walnuts
- 1/2 c. cornstarch
- 1 clove garlic
- 1 c. cooked quinoa
- 2 tbsp. canola oil
- 2 tsp. rice wine vinegar
- 3 green onions
- 4 medium portobello mushroom caps (about 1 lb.)

Whole-grain burger buns
- Sprouts
- Lettuce
- Sliced tomatoes
- For Rosemary Mayo
- 1/2 c. mayonnaise
- 1 tsp. finely chopped fresh rosemary
- 1 tsp. lemon juice
- Kosher salt

What to do first:
- Chop the red and the green onion
- Remove gills and chop Portobello mushroom caps
- Chop the fresh rosemary finely

Now for the Burgers:
- Preheat the oven to 375 degrees F
- Toss mushrooms with walnuts, garlic, 1 tablespoon oil, 3/4 teaspoon salt, and 1/4 teaspoon pepper; spread in even layer in a 3-quart, shallow baking dish

- Bake for 20 minutes or until mushrooms are tender
- Set aside to cool. Turn oven off.
- Pulse mushroom mixture, red onion, green onions, and vinegar until mostly smooth in a food processor scraping side of bowl if necessary
- Transfer the mixture to a large bowl and stir in quinoa and cornstarch until well-blended
- Cover bowl with plastic wrap and refrigerate for 2 hours
- Preheat the oven to 375 degrees F
- Line baking sheet with foil
- Form mixture into 5 patties (about 1/2" thick and 3" wide)
- In a 12" nonstick skillet, heat remaining 1 tablespoon oil on medium
- In 2 batches, cook patties 5 minutes or until well-browned, turning over once
- Transfer seared patties to prepared baking sheet
- Bake 10 minutes or until hot in centers

Next is for the Rosemary Mayo:
- Combine the following:
- Mayonnaise
- Rosemary
- Lemon juice
- A pinch of salt
- Serve burgers on buns with Rosemary Mayo, garnish with sprouts, lettuce, and tomato

Green Mushroom & Orzo Soup

What you need:
- 1/4 tsp. Kosher salt
- 1/4 c. garlic
- 1/2 c. shallots
- 1 c. sliced mushrooms
- 1 c. orzo
- 1 1/4 c. celery
- 2 tbsp. extra-virgin olive oil
- 3 c. broccoli
- 3 c. sliced spinach
- 8 c. vegetable or chicken broth
- basil pesto

Now for the main dish:
- Heat olive oil on medium in an 8-quart saucepot
- Add salt, celery, shallots, and garlic. Cook 8 minutes or until golden, stir.
- Add broth and broccoli. Heat to simmering on high. Reduce heat to medium-low
- Simmer 15 minutes, stir occasionally
- Add spinach, mushrooms and orzo and simmer for 8 to 10 minutes or until starches and veggies are softened.
- Remove from heat. Stir in basil pesto to taste.

Avocado Mash Paired with BBQ Chickpea & Cauliflower Flatbread

What you need:
- 1 tbsp. extra-virgin olive oil
- 2 tbsp. lemon juice
- 2 ripe avocados
- 2 tbsp. roasted salted pepitas
- 4 flatbreads or pocketless pitas
- 12 oz. small cauliflower florets
- salt
- BBQ Chickpea "Nuts"
- Hot sauce, for serving

What to do first:
- Toast flatbreads or pocketless pitas

  Now for the main dish:
- Toss cauliflower with olive oil and 1/4 teaspoon salt on a large rimmed baking sheet
- Roast in 425 degree F in the oven for 25 minutes along with one-fourth recipe BBQ Chickpea "Nuts."
- Mash avocados with lemon juice and pinch salt and spread all over flatbreads
- Top with roasted cauliflower, chickpeas and pepitas
- Serve with drizzle of hot sauce

Squash and Lentil Stew

What you need:
* 1/2 tsp. ground cardamom
* 1 tbsp. fresh ginger
* 1 tbsp. vegetable oil
* 1 tsp. ground coriander
* 1 tbsp. cider vinegar
* 1 small butternut squash
* 1 lb. green lentils
* 2 medium shallots
* 5 c. packed baby spinach
* 6 c. chicken or vegetable broth

What to do first:
* Peel and chop finely the fresh ginger
* Peel and see butternut squash and cut it into 1 ½" chunks
* Slice shallots thinly

Now for the main dish:
* Cook shallots and ginger in oil 5 minutes or until shallots are golden in pressure-cooker pot on medium, stir
* Add coriander and cardamom; cook 1 minute, stir
* Add the squash, lentils, broth and 1/4 teaspoon salt.
* Cover, lock and bring up to pressure on high
* Reduce heat to medium-low
* Cook for 12 minutes. Release pressure by using quick-release function
* Stir in spinach, vinegar and 1/2 teaspoon each of salt and pepper

Smoky Black Bean Soup

What you need:
* 1/4 c. tomato paste
* 1 medium onion
* 1 c. frozen corn
* 1 1/2 tsp. ground cumin
* 2 tbsp. extra virgin olive oil
* 2 medium carrots
* 2 stalks celery
* 3 cloves garlic
* 3 c. lower-sodium vegetable or chicken broth
* 3 cans (15 oz. each) lower-sodium black beans
* Avocado chunks and cilantro leaves, for serving

What to do first:
* Chop onion and carrots
* Slice celery
* Crush garlic cloves with press
* Undrain black beans

Now for the main dish:
* Heat oil on medium-high in a 12-inch skillet
* Add the carrots, celery, and onion
* Cook for 6 to 8 minutes or until starting to brown, stir occasionally
* Add tomato paste, garlic and cumin.
* Cook and stir 1 to 2 minutes or until garlic is golden and tomato paste has browned
* Stir in 1/2 cup broth, scrape up any browned bits
* Transfer contents of skillet to 6- to 8-quart slow-cooker bowl along with beans, corn and remaining broth
* Cover and cook on High for 4 hours or Low for 6 hours

- Serve with avocado and cilantro

Nutty Edamame and Noodle Salad

What you need:
* 1/2 c. peanut butter
* 1/2 c. rice vinegar
* 1/2 tsp. salt
* 1/2 c. fresh cilantro
* 1 tbsp. Sriracha hot sauce, plus more for serving
* 1 pt. grape tomatoes
* 1 medium Granny Smith apple
* 2 tbsp. water
* 2 c. frozen corn
* 3 bags (8 oz. each) shirataki noodles
* 3 c. frozen shelled edamame
* 3 c. carrots

What to do first:
* Chop the fresh cilantro
* Cut the grape tomatoes in half
* Quarter and slice Granny Smith apple thinly
* Rinse and drain shirataki noodles
* Shred the carrots

Now for the main dish:
* Heat large saucepot water to boiling on high then add shirataki noodles, edamame and corn
* Boil for 2 minutes. Rinse and drain well
* Whisk the peanut butter, rice vinegar, Sriracha hot sauce, water, and salt in a large bowl
* Add the shredded carrots, tomatoes, apple, cilantro and noodle mixture
* Toss until well coated
* Serve with Sriracha

Roasted Squash Mole Bowls

What you need:
* 1/2 c. raw shelled pumpkin seeds, plus more for garnish
* 1/2 tsp. cumin seeds
* 1/2 tsp. dried oregano
* 1/2 onion
* 1/2 c. coconut milk
* 1/2 c. parsley
* 1/4 c. packed cilantro, plus more for garnish
* 3/4 c. vegetable stock
* 1 jalapeno chile
* 1 large butternut squash
* 2 tomatillos
* 2 cloves garlic
* 3 tbsp. olive oil
* Lime wedges, for garnish
* Cooked rice, for serving

What to do first:
* Cut the onion into wedges
* Chop the parsley and cilantro
* Slice the jalapeno chile
* Peel and cut the butternut squash into 1" chunks
* Husk and half tomatillos
* Slice garlic cloves into halves

Now for the main dish:
* Preheat oven to 400 degrees F
* Toss the squash with 2 tablespoons olive oil, 1 teaspoon salt, and 1/4 teaspoon pepper
* Arrange on baking sheet; roast 35 to 40 minutes or until squash is tender, stir occasionally

- Meanwhile, toast pumpkin seeds, cumin seed and oregano in a 10" skillet on medium 3 minutes or until fragrant, stir
- Remove from heat; set aside.
- Heat the remaining 1 tablespoon olive oil on medium in the same skillet
- Add onion, tomatillos, garlic and jalapeno; cook 5 minutes or until slightly browned
- Place the vegetables, pumpkin seeds, and spice mixture in blender or food processor
- Pulse a few more times
- Add the following: coconut milk, cilantro, parsley, stock, 3/4 teaspoon salt, and 1/4 teaspoon pepper
- Process until smooth.
- Return the mixture in the skillet
- Simmer on medium heat and stir often for about 15 to 20 minutes or until slightly thickened
- Share out the rice and squash among 4 bowls; add some sauce
- Serve remaining sauce on the side, garnished with cilantro and lime wedges

Mixed Mushrooms in A Creamy Vegan Linguine

What you need:
- 1/4 c. nutritional yeast
- 1 lb. linguine or fettuccine
- 2 green onions
- 3 cloves garlic
- 6 tbsp. olive oil
- 12 oz. mixed mushrooms

What to do first:
- Slice green onions thinly on an angle
- Chop garlic cloves finely
- Slice mixed mushrooms thinly
- Now for the main dish:
- Cook linguine as label directs, reserving 3/4 cups pasta cooking water before draining. Return drained linguine to pot.
- Meanwhile, heat oil on medium-high in a 12" skillet
- Add the mushrooms and garlic; cook for 5 minutes or until mushrooms are browned and tender, stir
- Move it to the pot with the following: cooked, drained linguine, nutritional yeast, 1/2 teaspoon salt, reserved cooking water, and 3/4 teaspoon coarsely ground pepper
- Toss until well combined
- Garnish with green onions. Serve.

Crunchy Potatoes with Vegan Nacho Sauce

What you need:
*   1/4 c. nutritional yeast
*   1/2 jalapeno chile
*   1/2 tsp. chili powder
*   1/2 tsp. ground cumin
*   1/2 tsp. sweet paprika
*   1/2 tsp. garlic powder
*   1 tsp. Coarse sea salt
*   1 c. raw unsalted cashews
*   2 lb. mixed baby potatoes
*   3 tbsp. canola oil
*   3 tbsp. lemon juice

What to do first:
*   Seed and chop the jalapeno chile
*   Soak unsalted cashews overnight and drain
*   Cut the baby potatoes in halves

Now for the main dish:
*   Preheat oven to 450 degrees F. Toss potatoes with oil, 1/2 teaspoon salt, and 1/4 teaspoon pepper
*   Spread potatoes evenly on rimmed baking sheet; roast 30 minutes until golden and crispy, stir once
*   In the meantime, puree the following: cashews, chili powder, cumin, garlic powder, jalapeno, lemon juice, nutritional yeast, paprika, sea salt, and with 1 cup water in a blender until smooth
*   Bring the puree to a 2-quart saucepan
*   Heat it on medium-low for about 5 minutes or until warm, stir occasionally.
*   Transfer to bowl

- Serve with roasted potatoes
- Note: You can refrigerate remaining sauce up to 1 day. It is also good with tortilla chips, roasted cauliflower, and the like

Pumpernickel Panzanella with Garden Greens

What you need:
*   1/4 c. fresh dill
*   1/2 bunch watermelon or regular radishes
*   1 lb. asparagus
*   1 tbsp. white wine vinegar
*   1 tbsp. spicy brown mustard
*   1 tbsp. prepared horseradish
*   1 bunch green onions
*   2 tbsp. fresh lemon juice
*   2 tsp. extra-virgin olive oil, plus 2 Tbsp. for dressing
*   4 c. arugula
*   6 c. pumpernickel bread

*   What to do first:
*   Chop fresh dill
*   Trim and slice watermelon or regular radishes thinly
*   Trim and cut asparagus into 1" lengths
*   Prepare horseradish
*   Cut onions into 1" lengths
*   Cube pumpernickel bread about ¼"

*   Now for the main dish:
*   Arrange two oven racks in upper and lower thirds of oven
*   Preheat oven to 450 degrees F
*   Toss asparagus, green onions, 2 teaspoons olive oil, and 1/4 teaspoon salt on a large rimmed baking sheet; spread in a single layer

36

- Bake on lower rack until vegetables are browned and tender, 15 minutes
- Arrange bread in single layer on another large rimmed baking sheet
- Bake on upper rack until crisp and dry, stir once; 10 to 12 minutes
- Meanwhile, whisk remaining 2 tablespoons oil, lemon juice, vinegar, mustard, horseradish, and 1/2 teaspoon salt in large bowl; stir in dill
- Toss bread cubes with vinaigrette in bowl; add roasted vegetables, arugula, and radishes; toss until well-
- combined

Asparagus and Shiitake Tacos

What you need:
- 1/2 tsp. Kosher salt
- 1 tsp. ground chipotle chile
- 1 bunch green onions, trimmed
- 1 c. homemade or prepared guacamole
- 3 tbsp. canola oil
- 4 garlic cloves, crushed with press
- 8 oz. shiitake mushrooms, stems discarded
- 8 corn tortillas, warmed
- Lime wedges
- cilantro sprigs
- Hot sauce, for serving
- What to do first:
- Trim green onions
- Crush garlic cloves with a press
- Discard stems from shiitake mushrooms
- Warm tortillas

Now for the main dish:
- Heat grill on medium. Combine oil, garlic, chipotle, and salt in a large baking dish.
- Add asparagus, shiitakes, and green onions; toss to coat
- Grill asparagus until tender and lightly charred, turn occasionally; 5 to 6 minutes
- Grill shiitakes and green onions until lightly charred, turn occasionally; 4 to 5 minutes
- Transfer vegetables to cutting board
- Cut asparagus and green onions into 2" lengths and slice shiitakes
- Serve with corn tortillas, guacamole, lime wedges, cilantro, and hot sauce

Bulgur Pilaf with Garbanzos and Dried Apricots

What you need:
- ¼ c. fresh parsley leaves
- ½ c. Dried apricot
- ½ tsp. salt
- ¾ c. water
- 1 clove garlic
- 1 can garbanzo beans (chickpeas)
- 1 can vegetable broth or chicken broth
- 1 c. bulgur
- 1 tbsp. olive oil
- 1 small onion
- 2 tsp. curry powder

Now for the main dish:
- Heat water and 1 1/4 cups vegetable broth to boiling on high in a 2-quart covered saucepan
- Stir in bulgur; heat to boiling
- Reduce heat to medium-low; cover and simmer 12 to 15 minutes or until liquid is absorbed
- Remove saucepan from heat. Uncover and fluff bulgur with fork to separate grains
- Meanwhile, heat oil on medium in a 12-inch nonstick skillet, 1 minute
- Add onion and cook for 10 minutes, stir occasionally
- Stir in curry powder and garlic; cook 1 minute
- Stir in garbanzo beans, apricots, salt, and remaining 1/2 cup vegetable broth; heat to boiling
- Remove saucepan from heat; stir in bulgur and parsley

Black Bean Lasagna with No Cheese

What you need:
- ¼ tsp. garlic powder
- ¼ c. raw cashews
- ¼ c. nutritional yeast (optional)
- 1 can fire-roasted diced tomatoes
- 1 can tomato paste
- 1 c. water
- 1 small onion
- 1 tsp. dried oregano
- 2 can black beans
- 2 tbsp. finely chopped fresh basil
- 3 tbsp. olive oil
- 8 oz. no-boil lasagna noodles
- 14 oz. extra-firm tofu

Now for the main dish:
- Place tofu between 4 paper towel sheets. Place heavy skillet on top for 1 hour to press down on tofu
- Meanwhile, preheat oven to 375 degrees F. Into 4-quart saucepot, stir black beans, tomatoes, tomato paste, water, onion, oregano, garlic powder, 2 teaspoons salt, and 1/2 teaspoon pepper
- Heat to boiling on medium-high, stirring often. Reduce heat to maintain simmer; simmer, uncovered, 30 minutes, stir occasionally
- While the sauce cooks, pulse cashews until finely ground; transfer to large bowl, along with pressed tofu in food processor
- Crumble tofu using hands until texture resembles ricotta cheese

- If using yeast, stir it in along with the following: basil, olive oil, 1/4 teaspoon salt, and 1/8 teaspoon pepper
- Spread 1 cup tomato sauce and tofu mixture in a 13-by 9-inch glass or ceramic baking dish; repeat layering twice
- Top with 1 cup sauce. Spread sauce to completely cover noodles
- Bake, uncovered, 40 minutes or until noodles are tender
- Let it stand 15 minutes before serving

Moroccan Couscous Stew for Vegans

What you need:
- ⅓ c. golden raisins
- ¼ tsp. pie spice
- ½ c. vegetable broth
- 1 can stewed tomatoes
- 1 can chickpeas
- 1 tsp. ground cumin
- 1 c. vegetable broth
- 1 c. couscous
- 1 c. shredded carrots
- 1 zucchini
- 2 tsp. olive oil
- 2 tsp. Sriracha hot sauce
- 4 green onions

Now for the main dish:
- Heat 1 cup vegetable broth, in 1-quart saucepan, to boiling. Remove from heat; stir in couscous
- Cover; let stand 5 minutes
- Meanwhile, heat olive oil on medium in 12-inch nonstick skillet
- Add zucchini; cook 6 minutes, stir
- Add shredded carrots, green onions, golden raisins, ground cumin, and pie spice
- Cook 2 minutes, stir
- Add in stewed tomatoes, chickpeas, Sriracha hot sauce, and remaining 1/2 cup vegetable broth; break up tomatoes using a spoon
- Simmer 6 minutes or until tender. Serve stew over couscous.

Red Lentil and Veggie Soup

What you need:
*   1/8 tsp. ground black pepper
*   1/4 tsp. salt
*   1 bag baby spinach
*   1 tbsp. olive oil
*   1 small onion
*   1 tsp. ground cumin
*   1 can diced tomatoes
*   1 can vegetable broth
*   1 c. dried red lentils
*   4 medium carrots

Now for the main dish:
*   Heat oil on medium until hot in a 4-quart saucepan.
*   Add carrots and onion, cook for 6 to 8 minutes or until lightly browned and tender. Stir in cumin; cook 1 minute
*   Add the tomatoes, broth, lentils, 2 cups water, salt, and pepper; cover and heat to boiling on high
*   Reduce heat to low and simmer, covered, wait for 8 to 10 minutes or until lentils are tender
*   Stir in spinach. Makes about 7 1/2 cups

Beets and Greens Spaghetti

What you need:
- 1 tsp. salt
- 1 package spaghetti
- 2 bunch beets with tops
- 2 cloves crushed with garlic press
- 3 tbsp. olive oil
- 13 crushed red pepper

Now for the main dish:
- Cut tops from beets; reserve. If beets are inconsistent in size, cut the larger beets in half
- Place the beets and 1/2 cup water in deep 3-quart microwave-safe baking dish
- Cover and cook the beets in a microwave oven on High for around 15 to 20 minutes or until the beets are tender when pierced with tip of a fork or knife.
- Rinse the beets under cold running water until cool enough to handle
- Peel the beets and cut into 1/2-inch pieces
- Meanwhile, prepare spaghetti in boiling salted water as label directs in large saucepot
- Trim stems from beet tops. Coarsely chop beet greens; set greens aside
- Heat oil, garlic, and crushed red pepper in a nonstick 12-inch skillet over medium heat for 5 minutes or until garlic is lightly golden
- Increase heat to medium-high; add beet greens to skillet, and cook for 3 minutes, stir
- Add cooked beets and 1 teaspoon salt, and cook for 1 to 2 minutes or until mixture is heated through
- Remove 3/4 cup pasta cooking water when spaghetti has cooked to desired doneness
- Drain spaghetti and return to saucepot

- Add the beet mixture and reserved pasta cooking water; toss well

Acorn Squash with White Beans and Sage

What you need:
- ¼ tsp. salt
- ¼ tsp. coarsely ground black pepper
- ¾ c. vegetable broth
- 1 tbsp. olive oil
- 1 onion
- 1 medium carrots
- 1 can white kidney beans (cannellini)
- 1 medium tomato
- 2 clove garlic
- 2 small acorn squashes
- 3 tsp. fresh sage leaves
- Fresh sage sprigs for garnish
- Grated Parmesan cheese (optional)

Now for the main dish:
- Heat oil over medium-high heat until hot in a nonstick 12-inch skillet
- Add onion, carrot, and garlic, and cook for 15 minutes or until vegetables are tender and golden, stir occasionally
- Add the following: broth, beans, salt, pepper, and the 2 teaspoons of chopped sage
- Heat to boiling and cover skillet, keep warm
- Meanwhile, cut each squash lengthwise in half and remove seeds and strings
- Place squash halves in 3-quart microwave-safe baking dish
- Cover and cook the squash in a microwave oven on High for about 6 to 8 minutes or until squash is fork-tender
- Place squash halves, cut side up, on platter. Fill each half with one-fourth of bean mixture; sprinkle

with diced tomato and remaining 1 teaspoon
chopped sage.

- Garnish with sage springs. Serve with Parmesan if
desired.

Banana Berry Smoothie

What you need:
- ¼ cup low-fat granola
- ¼ cup blueberries, raspberries, blackberries, or strawberries
- ½ cup pomegranate, cherry, blueberry, or cranberry juice
- ½ cup low-fat plain or vanilla soymilk
- 1 cup blueberries, raspberries, blackberries, or strawberries
- 1 cup frozen unsweetened sliced peaches
- 1 cup ice cubes
- 1 medium banana, cut up

Here's what to do:
- Combine banana, 1 cup berries, peaches, fruit juice, and soymilk in a blender
- Cover and blend until smooth.
- Add ice cubes, one at a time, through the opening in the lid until combined and slushy with the motor running
- Top each serving with granola and ¼ cup berries

Baked Pumpkin with Cinnamon

Here's what you need:
- ¼ cup packed brown sugar
- ½ teaspoon salt
- 1 teaspoon ground cinnamon
- 2 tablespoons roasted peanut oil, peanut oil, cooking oil, or melted butter
- 3 pounds baking pumpkin or winter squash (butternut or acorn), peeled, seeded

What to do first:
- Peel and seed the pumpkin or winter squash

Here's what to do:
- Preheat oven to 325°F. Line a 3-quart rectangular baking dish with foil.
- Stir together brown sugar, cinnamon, and salt in a small bowl; set aside
- In the prepared 3-quart rectangular baking dish, toss pumpkin with oil
- Sprinkle brown sugar mixture evenly over pumpkin
- Bake, covered with foil, for about 40 minutes
- Uncover and stir pumpkin
- Bake, uncovered, for about 15 minutes more or until pumpkin is tender

Roasted Sweet Potatoes with Spicy Thai Peanut Sauce and Rice

Here's what you need:
- Spicy Thai Peanut Sauce
- ¼ cup reduced-sodium tamari or soy sauce
- ¼ teaspoon red pepper flakes
- ½ cup creamy peanut butter
- 1 teaspoon fresh ginger
- 2 tablespoons water
- 2 cloves garlic
- 2 tablespoons honey (or agave nectar, to taste)
- 3 tablespoons apple cider vinegar

Roasted Vegetables
- ¼ teaspoon cumin powder
- 1 red bell pepper
- about 2 tablespoons coconut oil (or olive oil)
- 2 sweet potatoes
- Sea salt, to taste

Rice and garnishes
- 1 ¼ cup jasmine brown rice (or any variety of long-grain brown rice)
- 2 to 3 green onions/chives
- Handful cilantro
- Handful peanuts
- Sriracha/rooster sauce on the side (optional)

Here's what to do first:
- Grate the fresh ginger
- Press garlic cloves
- Core, deseed, and slice red bell pepper into bite-sized strips

- Peel and slice potatoes into 1 inch long and 1/2 inch wide
- Slice the green onions/chives into thin rounds
- Torn the cilantro
- Crush the peanuts

Now for the main dish:
- Bring a large pot of water to boil
- Preheat the oven to 425 degrees Fahrenheit with a rack in the middle and another rack near the top
- Now, it's time to roast the vegetables:
- Heave the sweet potato chunks with a tablespoon of coconut oil, the cumin, and a sprinkle of salt
- Toss the bell pepper with about a teaspoon of coconut oil and salt. The vegetables should be lightly coated with oil on all sides
- In a single layer on a large baking sheet, arrange the sweet potatoes
- On a separate, smaller baking sheet, arrange the red bell peppers
- Roast the sweet potatoes on the middle rack for about 35 minutes, tossing halfway, and roast the peppers on the top rack for about 20 minutes, tossing halfway
- Cook the rice: Pour in the rice and give it a stir once the water is boiling
- Boil the rice for 30 minutes, then turn off the heat and drain the rice
- Return the rice to the pot and cover the pot
- For around 10 minutes, let the rice steam that way
- Remove the lid, fluff the rice with a fork and season with salt to taste
- Make the sauce: Whisk together the sauce ingredients in a bowl. If the sauce is too thick or too spicy, whisk in a little more water

- Lastly, top rice with roasted vegetables, a heavy drizzle of sauce, and a sprinkle of chopped green onions, cilantro and peanuts.
- Serve.

Banana Bread for Vegans

Here's what you need:
*   1/2 teaspoon kosher salt
*   1/2 cup plain soy milk yogurt
*   1/2 cup vegetable oil
*   3/4 cup sugar
*   1 teaspoon baking soda
*   1 teaspoon pure vanilla extract
*   1 1/4 cups unbleached all-purpose flour
*   3 very ripe medium mashed bananas, mashed (about 1 1/4 cups)
*   Cooking spray

Here's what to do:
*   Preheat the oven to 350 degrees F
*   Line the bottom and two long sides of a 9x5x3-inch loaf pan with parchment, leaving a 2-inch overhang on each long side, and lightly coat with cooking spray
*   Whisk the flour, baking soda and salt together in a medium bowl.
*   Whisk the bananas, sugar, yogurt, oil and vanilla together in another medium bowl
*   Using a rubber spatula, gently fold the wet ingredients into the dry ingredients until the batter comes together
*   Transfer the batter to the prepared loaf pan and bake until a tester inserted in the center comes out clean, for around 55 to 60 minutes; tent the loaf with foil if it is browning too quickly
*   For around 30 minutes, cool the loaf in the pan on a wire rack and lift it from the pan by the parchment overhangs
*   Cool completely on the rack

- Store the loaf in an airtight container at room temperature for up to 5 days

Meringue for Vegans

What you need:
- One 15-ounce can chickpeas
- 1/4 teaspoon cream of tartar
- Kosher salt
- 3/4 cup superfine sugar
- 1 large pastry bag
- 1 large star or round pastry tip

Here's what to do:
- Preheat the oven to 250 degrees F. Line 2 baking sheets with parchment.
- Strain the chickpeas directly into the bowl of a stand mixer. There must be about 3/4 cup liquid (reserve the chickpeas for another use)
- Add the cream of tartar and a pinch of salt to the liquid, and beat on medium-high speed until very foamy
- Add the sugar, 1 tablespoon at a time, while still beating, continue to beat until the mixture forms stiff and glossy peaks, for about 4 minutes
- Transfer the mixture to a large pastry bag fitted with a large star or round tip, and pipe 2-inch mounds about 2 inches apart onto the prepared baking sheets
- Bake until the meringues are set and no longer glossy, for about 2 hours, rotating the trays (from top to bottom) halfway through
- Turn the oven off, and let the meringues sit in the closed oven until they have dried out inside, for about 1 hour more.

Yummy Vegan Pancakes

What you need:
- 1/3 cup virgin coconut oil, melted
- 1 teaspoon pure vanilla extract
- 1 tablespoon baking powder
- 1 1/2 cups unsweetened plain soy milk
- 2 cups all-purpose flour
- 3 tablespoons sugar
- 4 teaspoons vegetable oil
- Fine salt
- Maple syrup, nut butter or jam, for serving

Here's what to do:
- Preheat the oven to 250 degrees F
- Whisk together the flour, sugar, baking powder and 1 teaspoon salt in a medium bowl
- Whisk together the soy milk, coconut oil and vanilla in a second medium bowl
- Add the soy milk mixture to the flour mixture and gently fold until just combined
- Over medium-low heat, heat a nonstick griddle or a large nonstick skillet
- Add 1 teaspoon of the vegetable oil
- Once the pan is hot, add three 1/4-cup mounds of batter, evenly spaced, and cook until the pancakes begin to bubble and are golden brown, for about 4 to 5 minutes
- Carefully flip the pancakes and cook until the underside is golden brown and the pancakes are cooked through, for around 3 to 4 minutes (adjust the heat as necessary for consistent browning)
- Do the same procedure with remaining batter and vegetable oil

- Don't forget to transfer the cooked pancakes in the oven to keep them warm
- Serve 2 per person with maple syrup, nut butter, jam or any of your favorite topping

Fruit and Almond Shortbread Bars

Here's what you need:
- 1/4 teaspoon kosher salt
- 1/2 cup sugar
- 1/2 teaspoon pure vanilla extract
- 1/2 teaspoon almond extract
- 1/2 cup white rice flour
- 1/2 cup potato starch
- 1 cup almond flour
- 1 cup fruit preserves
- 2 sticks (1 cup) vegan butter or margarine
- Sliced almonds, for topping

Here's what to do:
- Preheat the oven to 350 degrees F
- Grease an 8-inch or 9-inch square pan of your choice
- Beat the vegan butter and sugar until light and fluffy using a hand or stand mixer,
- Add the vanilla and almond extracts
- Mix the flours, starch, and salt in a medium bowl
- Add the dry ingredients to the "butter" mixture and mix until just mixed
- Press two-thirds of the dough into the pan and bake for about 10 minutes, or until the crust is pale light brown. Remove it from the oven when done
- Spread the preserves evenly over the crust when the pan has cooled enough to handle
- Break the remaining dough into little tiny pieces and drop them evenly over the jam. Top it off with the almonds
- Bake for another 25 to 30 minutes, or until the top is a nice golden brown
- Cut into bars and serve!

About the Author

The Health Buff is a group of writers that aims to help people on what diet they want to achieve. They explore a lot of dishes from different parts of the world and share them by putting everything into a book. These writers specifically share the diets and food that just actually worked for them.

The Health Buff writers are all food and health enthusiasts, thus, coming up with the idea of sharing what they all love to do to inspire other people look after their health. They all believe that the best investment that you can ever make is in your own HEALTH.